ISBN 978-1-62806-372-1 (print | paperback)

Cover layout by Salt Water Media
Interior layout by Morgan Stoevener, images used with the Canva License

Published by Salt Water Media
29 Broad Street, Suite 104
Berlin, MD 21811
www.saltwatermedia.com

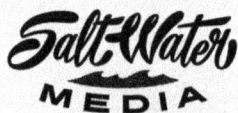

Salt Water
MEDIA

Welcome!

Welcome to CREATING YOUR JOURNEY, a companion guide for Riders of a Certain Age. I am thrilled that we are on this journey together! I'm Fran Severn, and I am delighted to be your guide.

We are starting a process together that will take us on a journey into your own personal dreams of horses, horseback riding, and just the joy of having horses in your life. Whatever your dreams are, you will be empowered to make them real in your life!

You may be a lady who once dreamed of horses and never got to have them in your life until now!

Or you may be someone who rode when you were MUCH younger but had to set horses aside for a while. Now you are returning, beginning again, and excited about rediscovering that joy.

Or you may be a lifelong horse person who is now exploring how horses will fit into your life as it changes, as you enter the realm of Riders of a Certain Age. What number you attach to that certain age is up to you. But whatever it is, aging with horses offers exciting opportunities and unique challenges.

This companion guide will help you question and explore this adventure. How it enhances your journey is entirely up to you.

So, are you ready to begin your journey?

Say YES!! Say YES!!
Here we go!

Fran

Introduction

I've designed this to be just what you need, when you need it. This is an interactive journey. You can go to any section of this guide and record just what you need.

I've built lots of help for you; think of it as the maps, rest areas, and guide to good places to eat along your journey.

You can find support in the book Riders of a Certain Age, at the companion website www.ridersofacertainage.com where you will find tons of information, and by joining the Riders Of A Certain Age Facebook Page: www.facebook.com/groups/ridersofacertainage

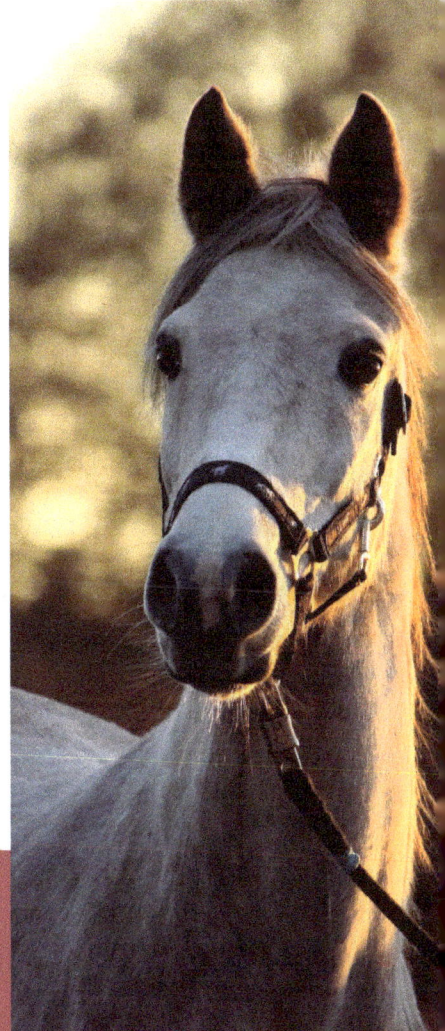

"The Sisterhood of horsewomen is unlike any other sorority I know. We bond through love of our horses and know that anyone who loves her horse is somene worth having in our lives."

~Fran Severn
Riders Of A Certain Age

TRACK YOUR PROGRESS

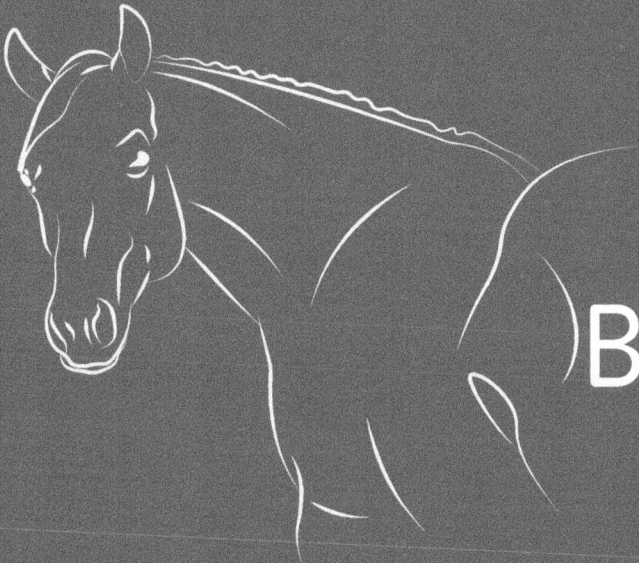

Before
Beginning

PREFACE

Have you ever noticed that the best part is the part before the first part?

It's kind of like the trailer for the movie. You watch it, enthralled. Even if you don't get what the movie is all about, you get an appetizer. A sneak peak. The trailer sets the tone for the movie. It introduces the characters and gives you a bird's eye view into their motivation or their situation.

In a book, the part before the first part is called the preface. Writing the preface for Riders of a Certain Age was just pure fun because it was the lovely moment when I got to share my origin story with my tribe.

And my tribe is YOU!

Where did my love for horses come from?
What are my earliest memories of horses in my life?
What were the outward symptoms of my inner horse infection?

And then, how did my life take me away from this inner dream?
How did horses continue to touch my life, even from afar?
And what occurred to bring me back to my dreams of horses?
Who were the important horse people?
And more importantly, who were the horses that were part of my own horse journey?

You have the opportunity to know me through my story (yes, you can find it in the preface of Riders of a Certain Age). And I want to know yours!

Using the prompts from the previous page, write your loving horses origin story here:

_____

_____

_____

_____

_____

_____

_____

_____

_____

_____

_____

_____

_____

_____

_____

_____

This is where each of us begins our journey. The next chapters are ours to write as we choose.

GETTING THE MOST OUT OF CREATING YOUR JOURNEY

Throughout this companion guide there are questions for you to answer and prompts to help you organize your thoughts so that you can write your own personal journey. The document you create will guide your horse activities as you pass through this Certain Age. My wish for you is that this resource will bring you peace, that through it you will know that you "have dotted your I's" and "crossed your T's" so that you can just sit back and completely enjoy your horse and your horse-filled life.

Here are some tips and hints for success:
- The journey is best enjoyed when you can travel it with like minded folks, so sharing is important! Join the Facebook group www.facebook.com/groups/ridersofacertainage
- If you are comfortable with a computer, consider typing your answers and your plans in a Word document. That makes it easy to copy and paste when you want to share with your group.
- You will find that there are lines here in the companion guide that you can write by hand, or just print and tape it in. It's your creation! Use it any way that is easy for you.
- Collect photographs as you go along. Our modern-day cell phones make taking pictures simple and easy. Sharing them is a joy!
- Be ready to help each other. From time to time I will invite you to be part of an even larger community where your stories can reach other people. When that invitation comes, say YES!!

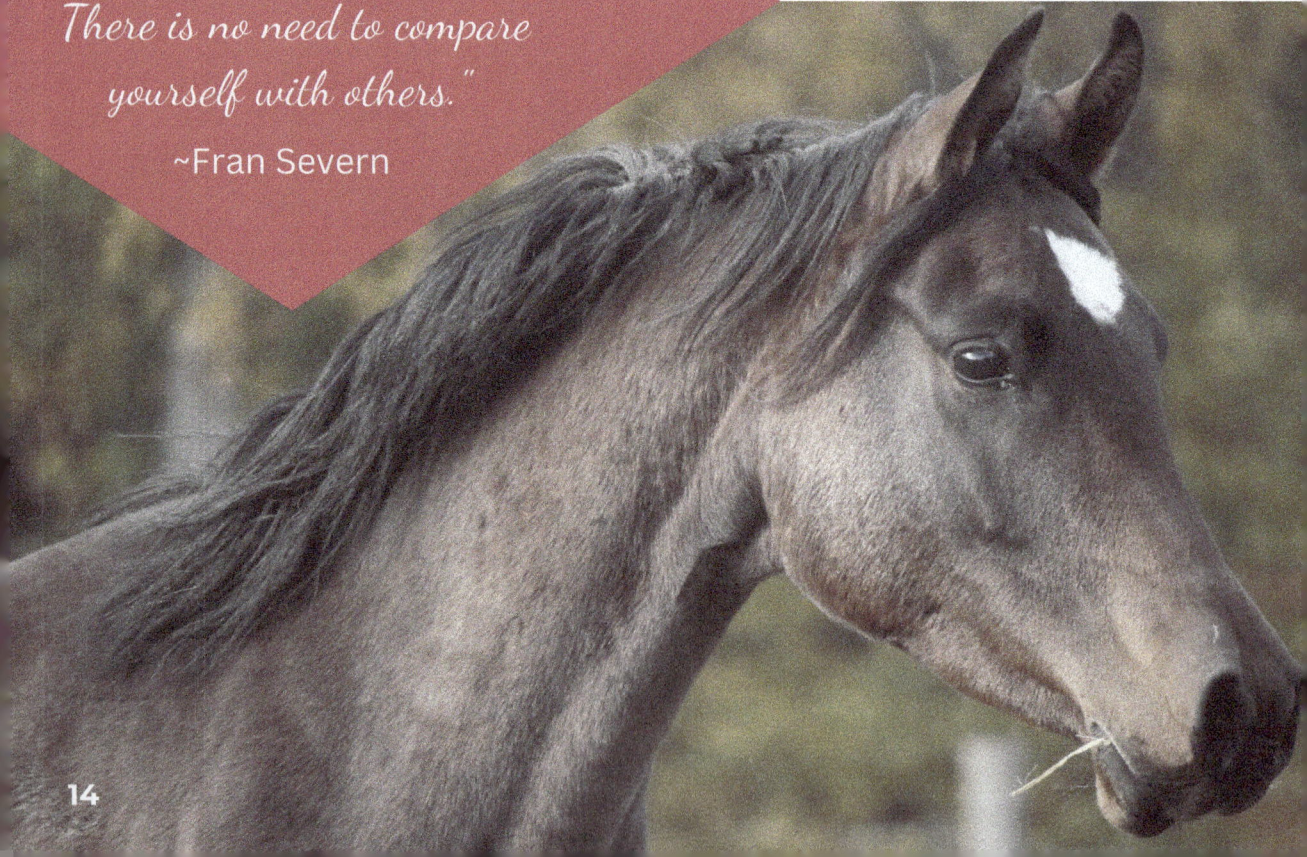

Remember that you don't have to have all the answers on your own. Check out the cool references in the back of Riders of a Certain Age.

If you don't yet own a copy of my book you can get one on the www.ridersofacertainage.com website. And there are also a lot of additional resources on the website.

"You are on your OWN path and journey. There is no need to compare yourself with others."

~Fran Severn

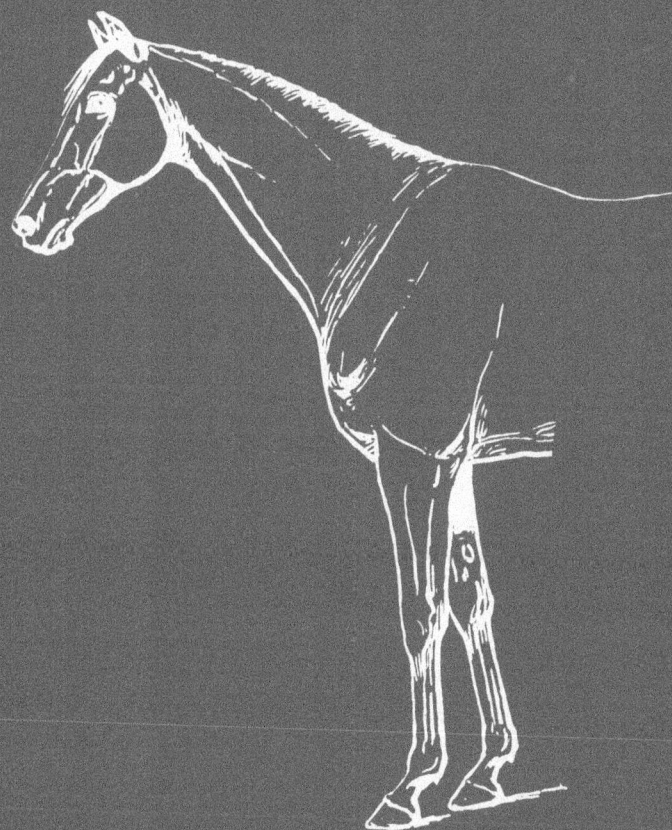

PART ONE

Getting
Started

WOMEN AND HORSES: WHY AND HOW WE LOVE THEM

Does your head swivel when you drive past a field of grazing horses?

Do you want Budwieser to bring back the ads with the Clydesdales?

Does a dude ranch vacation sound more appealing than a Caribbean Cruise?

YOU might be a horse person! You are not alone. About seven million Americans identify themselves as horse people.

What part of horses engages your heart:

Casual Trail Riding

Local horse shows

Hunt club

Gymkana and/or Rodeo

Breeding and raising babies

The Sport Horse disciplines: Dressage, Eventing, Hunters, or Jumpers

The Western Breed competitions: Quarter Horses, Appaloosas, Paints

The Other Breeds: Arabians, Pintos, Morgans and more

Racing and fractional ownership

Harness Racing

Polo

Western Dressage

Extreme Trail Courses or Competitive and Distance Trail Riding

Travel with my horse

OK, I can't list them all so share your own area of interest here.

_____

_____

_____

_____

_____

_____

_____

_____

_____

_____

_____

_____

_____

_____

_____

_____

While it's fun to identify our own personal area of interest with horses, it is even more significant to understand our own personal WHY.

What is the source of your attraction to horses?
There is plenty of research to help us discover why women are drawn to horses. You can read more about it in Chapter 1 of Riders of a Certain Age.

So what's your connection?
What does being around horses do to and for you?
How do you feel when you are near or riding a horse?
What is your earliest horse memory?

_____

_____

_____

_____

_____

_____

_____

_____

For many people "riding" is all about being on top of the horse. For others the horse represents a holistic relationship that is as significant for those who chose not to sit astride but to be in relationship with horses on the ground.

What is your own personal understanding of "Riding"?

What experiences of the horse are available to you on the ground?

What is your biggest source of satisfaction with your horse?

_____

_____

_____

_____

_____

Horses offer us both recreation and responsibilities.

What responsibilities are you ready to take on for your horse?

Which horse responsibilities are you just as happy to hand over to someone else?

_____

_____

_____

_____

_____

_____

Imagine all the ways the horses can offer you recreational activities.

Which sound like the most fun to you?

How about an ocean cruise with lots of fellow horse people? It's all the benefits of cruising with folks that think like you (unlimited horse conversation!)

How about an adventure of the Old West? You can ride the range and work cattle. You can discover western horse sports at the guest ranch. Some are as rustic as the Ponderosa while others are 4-star resorts with hot tubs in view of the pastures.

How about summer camp for adult riders (we call these retreats!) where you can combine a weekend of equine education with a great social experience in the company of other horse crazy ladies.

You can particiate in historical cavalry re-enactments of the Civil and Revolutionary Wars.

You can enjoy destination travel tours all over the world.

Share your dream recreational experience, one you have already enjoyed, or one you are dreaming of (hint: if you want to enjoy the dreaming process you can search up all kinds of equestrian travel opportunities online. The Resources section of the website lists many of them.)

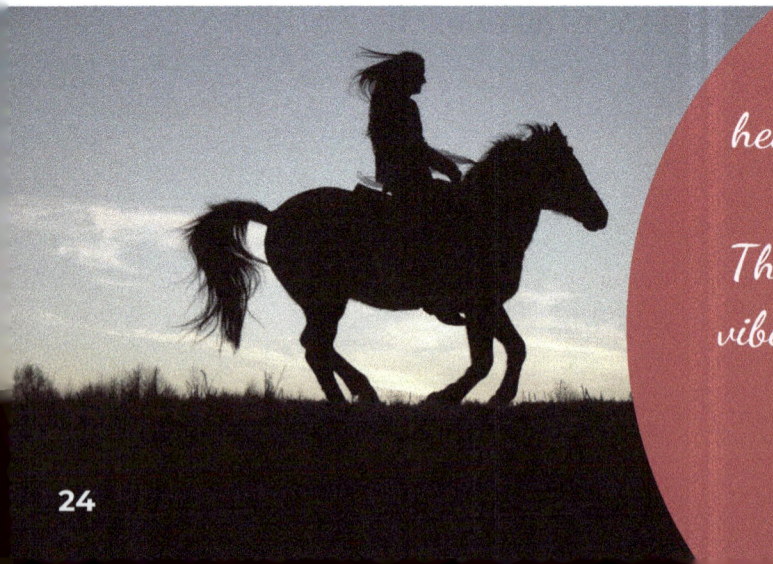

_____
_____
_____
_____
_____
_____
_____
_____

"A horse can hear a human heartbeat from 4 feet away. They hear intentions, feel vibes. They are mirrors of the soul."

~Fran Severn

FINDING AN INSTRUCTOR: IT'S LIKE LOOKING FOR THE PERFECT PARTNER

Remember that I said YOU are not alone? Now it's time to choose one of the most important sidekicks of your horse journey.

You have done enough dreaming to know your first goal. Share it here:

_____

_____

_____

_____

_____

_____

_____

The most significant helper for reaching your dreams and goals is your riding instructor.
Do you already have a riding instructor that you love and trust?

If yes, Congratulations!!

If not, it's time to get to work. You are looking for the person who fits you. One who meets your needs both in knowledge and personality, and who has access to the right facilities and horse teaching partners to help you reach your first goals.

Where can you look for instructors?
What riding groups are in your area?
What stables and riding schools?
What riding associations have chapters in your area?
What do you consider important qualities for your instructor to have?

What are the top five things that you are looking for in an instructor?

_____

_____

_____

_____

_____

_____

_____

What is your plan for getting to know your instructor candidates?

I'm going to call them and talk about my hopes and dreams.
I want them to propose a way for us to begin.
I will visit the barn.
I want to watch a lesson (for a rider like me) and learn where she is on her journey and how her instructor helps her.
I will explore the instructor's ability to work with any physical concerns that I have.
In order to facilitate a great conversation with your instructor candidate you need to be clear about your riding goals.
What do you want to get out of a lesson?
What is your immediate riding goal?
What is your long-term riding goal?
What do you look for at a riding stable?

MY PLAN FOR INTERVIEWING AN INSTRUCTOR

_____

_____

_____

_____

_____

_____

In your physical farm visit you can observe, and learn about the character of the learning environment as well as its content.

Use this tool , from Riders of a Certain Age by Fran Severn

"Lesson Barn Evaluation"

- Is the riding area prepared for lessons? Is all the equipment needed on hand and in place?

  _____

- Is the instructor focusing entirely on the lesson, or does she stop to deal with other barn issues, phone calls, and interruptions?

  _____

- Does she seem to enjoy teaching?

  _____

- Are the instructor and the student comfortable with each other?

  _____

- Is the instructor patient?

  _____

- Is she asking for feedback, encouraging questions, and striving to clarify things when the student is confused?

  _____

- Is she flexible in explaining concepts and how to do things?

  _____

"Lesson Barn Evaluation" Continued

- Short-tempered, sarcastic or belittling comments about the rider are a warning sign. Ditto if she makes snide remarks about other riders, trainers, or instructors.

_____

- How many days a week does she teach, and when?

_____

- Do you have a choice of group lessons, which are often less expensive, or private lessons? Many instructors want you to begin with private lessons so they can concentrate on teaching you the most important basics without distraction. Don't be put off by the prospect of riding with kids if that's an option. Their enthusiasm and joy are contagious.

_____

- If riding a lesson horse, will you ride the same horse for each lesson, or will you ride different ones?

_____

- If you already have a horse, will she ride and evaluate him? (She should want to do this so that she can learn his movements, quirks, and abilities.)

_____

"Lesson Barn Evaluation" Continued

- Is she willing to ride your horse at other times (for an additional fee, of course) to work on training elements that are beyond your abilities or time?

- Are you allowed to video lessons so you can review on your own? Seeing what you are doing makes it easier to transfer those concepts into the saddle. Not all stables have that ability, but it's becoming a common option with the popularity of sports camera devices and video apps.

- When is payment due? Are there pre-pay packages of four or five lessons, perhaps for a discount? This is a good option. You'll rarely be able to decide if an instructor is right for you after just one lesson. Ride several times at one place before trying another. It takes a few lessons to get comfortable with the instructor and the rhythm of the program.

- What are the cancellation policies? These often seem harsh. However, clients are notorious for canceling at the last moment or just not showing up at all, which is, at best, rude. No-shows mean no income. No instructor will retire to Barbados on her income from teaching lessons or running a boarding stable, so no-shows seriously damage her bottom line. As a result, they are strict about their payment plans.

"Lesson Barn Evaluation" Continued

- You know what to expect from your instructor; what can your instructor expect from you? You are building a relationship with a person who is your most important helper in Creating Your Journey with horses.

_____

_____

_____

_____

_____

_____

- What are the commitments you are making to your own learning journey?

_____

_____

_____

_____

_____

_____

Check out Chapter Two, the section on being a good student, in Riders of a Certain Age.

What makes a good student?

How can you show your lesson horse that you appreciate him?

How can you contribute to the positive ambiance of the riding stable?

What other commitments you are making to your own learning journey?

_____

_____

_____

_____

_____

_____

_____

"The moment I put my left foot in the stirrup, step up on the horse, and settle in the saddle, I just come alive. It's the greatest feeling in the world."

~Helen Crabtree

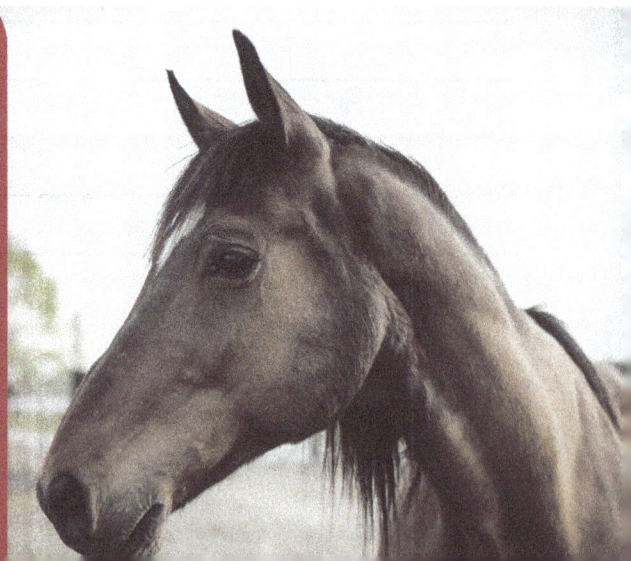

Remember that being of a Certain Age may translate to fears, limitations, and points of view that affect the way you learn. Having clear expectations of your own role in the learning process will make it easier to create your journey your way and on your timetable.

Do you find that you learn better from physical activity? Or from mental activity? Or a combination of both?

Is your memory still sharp? Or do you need to have some grace with yourself in this area?

Much of learning to ride is about developing specific body memory of things you have not done before. What is your own story of how your age impacts learning new and complex physical activities?

_____

_____

_____

_____

_____

_____

_____

_____

How you define your abilities and limitations will become your truth so take care with the language you use.

What happens if you live where there are no nearby instructors? What are your options?

You will be able to create your own learning plan with some of these elements:
- Home study courses
- Clinics, to participate and to audit
- Virtual Coaching/Video Coaching
- Self Directed Study
- Books, Videos, "How To" websites
- Podcasts and Webinars
- Social Media (check the credentials of the source)
- College and University programs, both mounted riding and horse husbandry

Now make your own plan:

_____

_____

_____

_____

_____

_____

_____

A STABLE ENVIRONMENT: THE PLACE, THE PEOPLE, AND YOU

Entering the horse world can be very confusing. It's not a retail or business setting where most companies are similarly organized. In the horse world, each stable, each riding school, and rach farm is unique.

And it's much more about service than it is about the product or even the facilities. In other words, it's all about the people. A stable's environment is created by the people who own the business, the people who run it, and the people who provide direct care for you and your horse.

What matters most is the fit of the business with you, your goals, your dreams, and your journey.

What kind of atmosphere are you looking for at your riding stable?

_____

_____

_____

_____

_____

_____

_____

_____

_____

What kind of activity interests you: Very busy? Lots of classes? Group or private lessons? Kids and parents? Adults only? Interested in competition? Social activities in addition to riding?

_____

_____

_____

_____

_____

_____

What are some of the barn rules?

It's handy to have a clear expectation of your own must haves and those things that are bonus points in looking for the right barn for you. How do each of these rate on your list?

A clean barn in good repair.
A minimum of clutter.
Reasonable cleanliness, a barn is not a house but it isn't a trash dump either.
Organized cleaning tools.
Secure storage bins.
Feed room out of reach for the horses.
Charts to show what the feed rations are for each horse.
Vet and Farrier schedules that are easy to understand.
A hang out space for clients, inside or outside the barn.
Notice board for barn communications.
Phone service.
Internet service.
Accessible fire extinguishers.
Security cameras.
A locked tack room when the barn is closed.
Organized tack room.
Saddles and bridles in good repair.

List Continued

Supplies neatly arranged.
Water hose neatly coiled.
Wash rack has hot water.
Washer-dryer on the premises.
Clean and neat rest rooms.
Sound system.
Student interaction with their assigned horses beyond the riding arena.
Horses that are kept in stalls are content.
Plenty of grass available in the fields.
Friendly herd with no aggressive horses.
Helmet guidelines.
Liability signage as required by law.

What are your barn must haves?

_____

_____

_____

_____

_____

_____

_____

Choosing a barn and living with one are sometimes very different. You may discover that the culture of the barn does not live up to its advertisement.

How do you deal with gossip and unfriendly people?

What is your "get along with others" plan?

MY "GET ALONG WITH OTHERS" PLAN

_____

_____

_____

_____

_____

_____

_____

_____

There are many reasons for moving barns. It can arise from a wish to progress beyond the scope of your present barn or try a different discipline. Or the barn schedule no longer works for you. You might have discovered things that you can't stand about your current barn. Maybe you found a new community to be part of. Or you are facing new financial constraints.

Searching for a new barn is just like searching for your first barn.

What would make you want to move to another barn?
How would you address this to the management of your current barn?
Are you ready to move immediately if you are asked to do so/ (This could be if there is a waiting list for your stall, not necessarily that there is bad blood about your wanting to leave.)

Put your plan to paper so that if the need arises you will not be caught off guard. It is best to act in advance so you don't need to react should the time come to leave. Plan matters in order to have a graceful exit and a smooth transition.

MY RELOCATION PLAN

_____

_____

_____

_____

_____

_____

WHAT TO WEAR: EQUINE FASHIONISTAS

Hey baby, you are looking good! Riding clothes that work really matter.

The basics are a good pair of boots and a certified safety helmet. Don't scrimp on these. Next comes your choice of leggings which is influenced by your riding discipline. Jeans work best for all the western disciplines and breeches for the sport horses.

You can fashion your riding wardrobe to reflect your own style. And on the practical side always dress for the weather.

What sort of clothing do you need for the riding that you do?

MY CLOTHING CHECKLIST

_____

_____

_____

_____

_____

_____

Where are the best places to look for the clothing, if it is not available at a store nearby? (Hint: A list of current online retailers is on the website.)

_____

_____

If you wish to add competition to the games you play with horses then ask your riding instructor or coach for a specific list. They will have very specific guidelines and since competition clothing is expensive it is wise to seek the exact standards they recommend.

MY COMPETITION CLOTHING PLAN

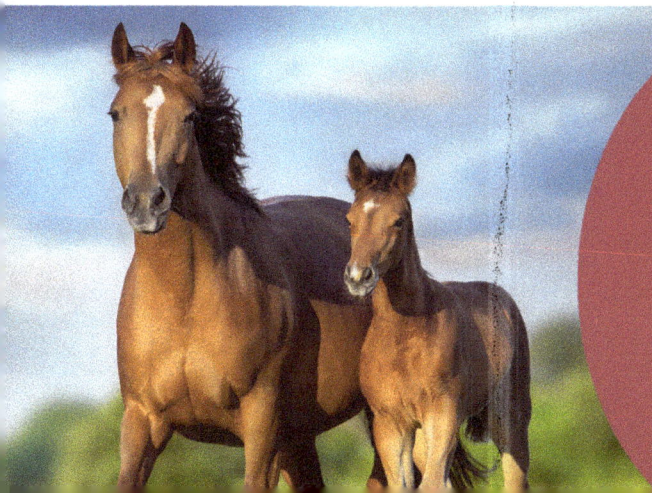

_____

_____

_____

_____

"Dumping money into your hobby is investing in your passion. Never let anyone undermine your hobbies."

~Fran Severn

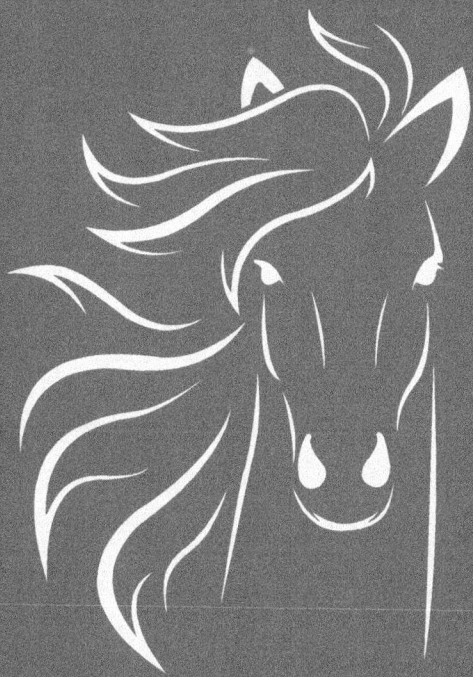

PART TWO

Fitness And The Rider Of A Certain Age

EASING INTO THE SADDLE: KNOWING WHAT YOU CAN DO

As Riders, we expect our horses to be physically fit and able to do what we ask with power and ease. For many riders the sense that this power, the horse's power, available to us is part of the draw, the dream of horses. With a horse we are more than ourselves.

In a world where women struggle at all ages and stages of life with concerns about being enough, with our horse we are whole.

Yet few of us really expect as much in our own physical preparation as we expect of our horse. Even if we were once athletically fit as we age it becomes more and more difficult to keep up our conditioning.

The first step is figuring out what we can do and what limitations we have, what accommodations need to be made. Begin with a baseline.

How would you describe your current level of fitness?
Are you flexible?
How much stamina do you have?
How strong are you?
When was your last physical check-up?
What are your hidden physical concerns about riding?

MY BASELINE

———————————————
———————————————
———————————————
———————————————
———————————————
———————————————
———————————————

GETTING FIT: TRAINING, TRAINERS, AND THERAPIES

Sue Cumming Schultz, whose students have won over 850 National and World Championships, comes to lead a clinic. She picks up a marker and writes the first maxim of the day on the board: **Expect twice as much of yourself as you do of your horse.**

Sue is one of the great training minds of the horse industry. A multiple World and National Champion trainer in her own right, she is committed to constant and continuing education and in serving the whole horse community. Fairly early in her professional career she experienced extreme vertigo, a condition caused by the overdevelopment of muscles in her shoulders, neck and back that developed from riding.

Her doctors declared an end to her own riding career because it so severely damaged her health. She was forced to a new path, forced to transition from active riding to teaching and coaching. Yet in order to continue her physical pursuit of greatness she found a new way. She added yoga to her life and discovered all the ways that a new routine of both physical and mental preparation contributed to her skills with horses.

Even though we Riders of a Certain Age face unique physical challenges, this does not necessitate giving up on becoming our very best physical self in order to partner our horses. Each person will find her own way.

These prompts can help you:

What is your regular exercise routine?
What are you looking to accomplish with an exercise routine?
What options do you have for finding and working with a personal trainer?
What options do you have for online training?
What online apps and videos have you tried?
Do you think a fitness tracker can help you meet your goals? Why or why not?
What are the differences between Pilates, Yoga, Chiropractic, and Somatics?
Which of these might help you reach your fitness goals?

MY FITNESS PLAN

_____

_____

_____

_____

_____

_____

WEIGHT AND RIDING: A TOUCHY SUBJECT

One of the best exercises in compassion for our horses is to experience what it feels like to carry fifteen to twenty percent of your weight on your back for extended periods of time.

You could load a backpack up with thirty pounds of books, sling it up on both shoulder straps and walk, trot and canter around a sand arena for an hour. This is pretty much your horse's experience of you. One of our first goals as riders is to get skilled at our own self carriage so we do not burden our horse.

Our weight also contributes to our own risks while riding. Balance, flexibility, and posture are all influenced by weight.

How much we weigh, and what we do about maintaining a healthy weight matters to both us and to our horse.

MY HEALTHY WEIGHT PLAN

_____

_____

_____

_____

_____

_____

_____

Do you know what your optimum weight is?
How did you determine that?
How does being overweight affect your ability to ride comfortably and safely?
What are the safest and most effective ways to lose weight?
How much weight can you safely lose in a week?

FEAR: FORGET EVERYTHING AND RUN

There's an odd feature of the riding world: women love horses, but the desire to be with horses is often mixed with fear.

Your dreams are big and as long as they are only dreams they are safe. Then along comes reality, a reality you have craved so long that it seems almost inevitable that the fear is just around the corner. You imagine a horse that loves you and you have a horse that has his own agenda, his own fears, needs, and opinions.

You plan for your education and along the way you encounter challenges. You might not be the one falling off but the idea of it is overwhelming. You want it so much that you are caught unawares when your heart rate speeds up and you begin to sweat, and maybe the fear even results in tears.

These are real physical signs that fear is present and you can't just wish it away. More than that, you won't just wish your horse dreams away. They are here to stay. The fact that you continue to create your journey with horse is evidence that horses are addictive! We can't stay away.

This fear is a factor that you must plan for with a clear action plan (the cure for FEAR is action!).

What makes you afraid of being around horses?
What makes you afraid of riding?
How anxious are you when you ride?

Do you become more confident and comfortable the longer you ride?

Do you talk about this with your instructor or other people at the stable?
What do you do to try to relieve your fears?
Have you tried programs that teach ways to overcome your worries?
What other confidence building things have you heard of?
Have you tried any of them?

MY COURAGE IN THE FACE OF FEAR PLAN

_____

_____

_____

_____

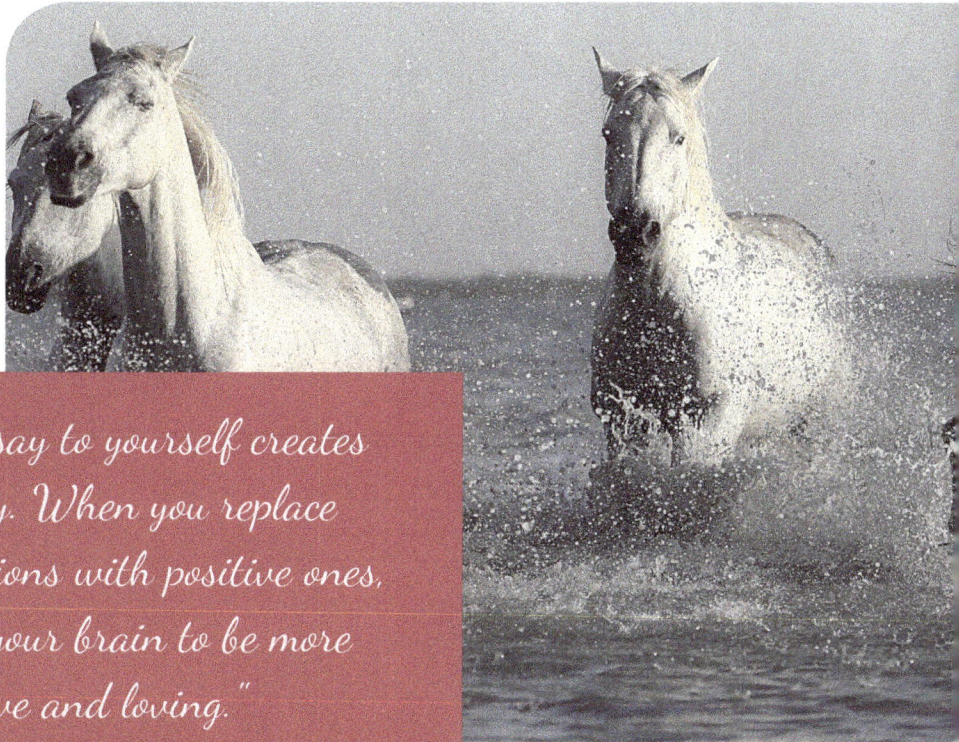

"What you say to yourself creates your reality. When you replace negative emotions with positive ones, you rewire your brain to be more positive and loving."

~Fran Severn

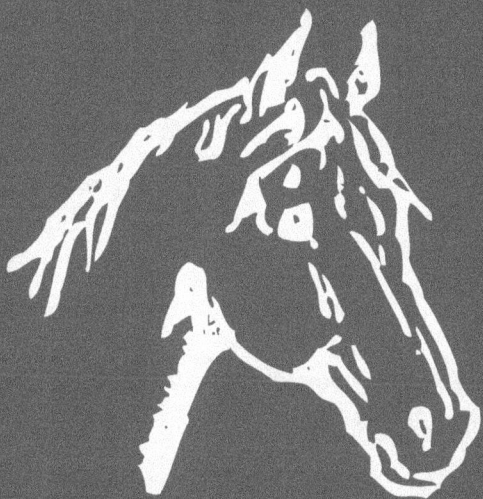

PART THREE

Safety And
The Rider Of
A Certain Age

PROTECTION AND PREVENTING INJURY: BALANCE, FALLS, VESTS, AND HELMETS

The number one action to take for your protection and to prevent injury is to be actively invested in your own rider education. Nothing is more valuable to your safety in riding than a continuing relationship with your riding instructor, trainer, and coach. They are the experts that help translate your horse's experience of you so that you can be an active participant in safety for both your horse and yourself.

As Roy Rogers said, "When you're young and fall off your horse, you may break something. When you are my age and you fall off, you splatter."

It's time to make a splatter resistant plan!

Since falls are a major concern as we age (and these falls may have nothing to do with your horse) we need to develop balance and core strength.

How balanced are you?

What do you do to maintain and improve your balance?

How do you measure your core strength?

What do you do to maintain and improve your core strength? (Hint: Strong core strength is vital for good riding.)

MY BALANCE AND CORE STRENGTH PLAN

_____

_____

_____

_____

What are the advantages of wearing a safety vest?

What sort of helmet do you wear?

What sort of medical alert or emergency device do you wear when you are at the stable or riding?

MY SAFETY EQUIPMENT PLAN

_____

_____

_____

_____

WHEN TO QUIT: QUESTIONS TO ASK AND OPTIONS

I've never met a lady whose dream of horse was "Now that I finally get to have horses in my life I think I'll quit in just a few years." for those of us who are Riders of a Certain Age, particularly if we are finally able to have horses, our dreams are infinite!

Do you see an end to your riding? Or are you riding off into the sunset?

We don't start into our horse life planning to quit. Yet for many of us the day will come for this consideration.

It may be a transition point. Like we move from riding astride as our primary joy to one of the unmounted relationships with horses. Whether a full stop or a gentle transition, as with everything planning makes it easier.

What factors in your decision as to whether to stop riding?
If you can no longer get into the saddle, what other options do you have?
What would you do to stay involved with horses if you could not get into the saddle?

MY TRANSITION PLAN

_____

_____

_____

_____

_____

_____

_____

PART FOUR

Uniquely Ours: Health Issues Kids Don't Face

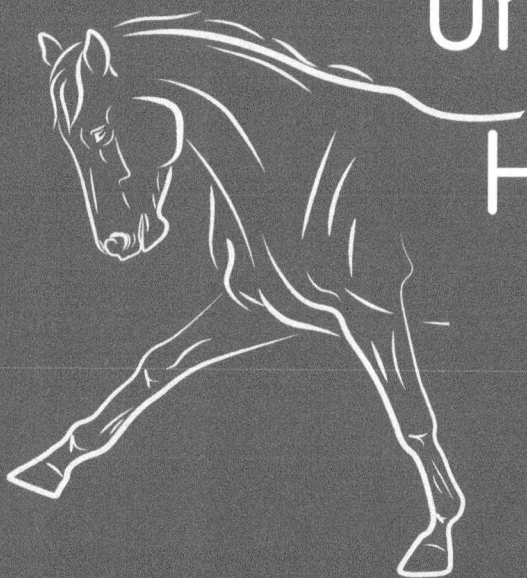

WHAT CHANGES WITH THE YEARS

Here we are, living our happy lives, reaching the apex of our career or enjoying retirement, spoiling our grandkids, indulging in our love of horses and *wham*, we start having medical problems. Very few of us would pass the pre-purchase exam we ask of our newly purchased horse. It's a simple truth. We change as we age.

Some of these changes are known. They come on gradually and we make adjustments to our lives When we add riding into our physical fitness equation we will face some challenges.

The good news is that few things we face will destroy our dreams. We just need a plan.

If you are dealing with menopause, how are you dealing with the symptoms?
When was your last bony density scan?
What are you doing to maintain or improve that condition?
How are you adjusting to a slower metabolic rate and (sadly) almost inevitable weight gain?

MY PERSONAL HEALTH PLAN: PART 1

_____

_____

_____

_____

BOUNCING, CHAFING, LEAKING, AND ARTHRITIS

As our body changes we need some support. For ladies this starts with creating comfort for "the Girls." Without proper support, riding can be uncomfortable!

Do you have undergarments that 'do their job' and fit?
If not, where are you looking for them?

MY "SUPPORT THE GIRLS" PLAN

_____

_____

_____

If you chafe, what have you tried to limit your discomfort?
Are you dealing with urinary incontinence?
Do you know the different types and causes?
Have you discussed the problem with a physician or nurse practitioner?
If you are dealing with arthritis, what actions are you taking?

MY PERSONAL HEALTH PLAN: PART 2

_____

_____

_____

_____

VISION, SLEEP, HEARING, AND BREATHING

Your horse is a creature of nature. Putting yourself inside his way of seeing and hearing and sleeping and breathing will contribute to you having a great relationship with him. To be equipped for this you need to tune up your own senses.

As we age one of the areas that dulls down is our own sensory perception. Our horses, meanwhile, are highly attuned to the natural world. The survival of the specie horse for the 65 million years of evolutionary development has relied on his ability to sense the natural world and respond immediately to any danger to him.

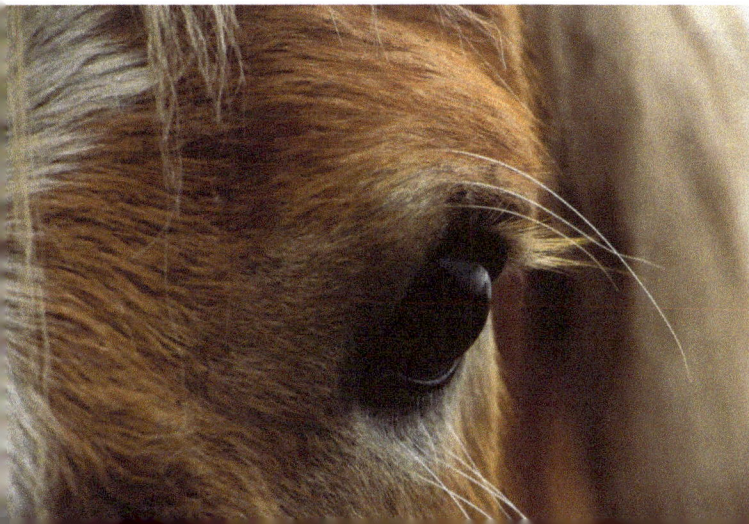

"Don't you dare let them tell you that you're too old or that it's too late. If you are still standing, then anything is possible."

~Fran Severn

Horses are highly developed prey animals, psychologically like deer. And we (yes, even we ladies) are apex predators. Taking good care of your sensory tools helps you be equipped to provide your horse with a safe life.

When was your last vision check-up?

What are the most common vision issues as we grow older?

How are you addressing them?

How many hours of 'quality sleep' do you get each night?

What are your strategies for getting enough sleep?

What are the most common hearing problems?

How much cardiovascular exercise do you get to improve your overall health and especially you lung capacity?

MY PERSONAL HEALTH PLAN: PART 3

_____

_____

_____

_____

PART FIVE

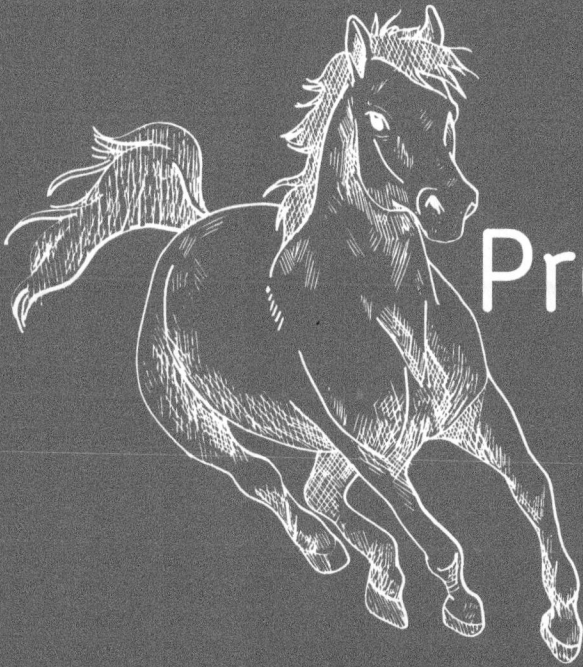

But He's So Pretty: Buying A Horse (Or Not)

SHOPPING FOR A HORSE: WHAT ARE YOU LOOKING FOR AND WHERE DO YOU FIND IT?

Congratulations! Shopping for a horse is like searching out a mate. Your riding education is designed to help you be ready for a long term relationship with your horse. You might find that you spend as much time with your horse as you do your spouse or family. And shopping for the horse is kind of like dating that leads to marriage!

So start with: What are you attracted to? Here are some prompts..

What are your favorite breeds of horses?
Why do you like those breeds?
What do you want to do with your horse?

This is my dream horse:

_____
_____
_____
_____
_____
_____

Now that you know what you are looking for, how will you go about finding it?

What are the advantages and disadvantages of buying or leasing?

_____

_____

_____

_____

_____

_____

_____

What is the most important bit of advice for horse-shoppers?

GET HELP!! Choosing the right mentor will lead you to the right horse. Without one your horse hunt may very well end in disaster.

Here is a story from my friend Deb Dyer (a professional trainer and riding coach)..

"I was at a horse show with several young ladies who were at the beginning of their interest in showing. One of the Moms came and asked me a question...

She said, "Do you know the difference between a good horse and a bad horse just by looking at them? Because they are all so pretty to me."

I chuckled and replied, "Yes, I do. Imagine that you are an alien from outer space and you land your ship in the middle of the CarMax parking lot. You would look around at all the pretty cars and have no idea the value of any of them because they are all painted up pretty and shiny. This is what it is like to shop for a horse when you don't know how to check out the mechanics, what is under the hood."

The right mentor knows how to look beneath the surface of the horse and see the parts that are critical for you to have a good horse partner. Your horse will uniquely fit your needs if you get good guidance from a mentor.

Who can you ask to help you find a horse?
What are your mentor's recommendations on shopping for your horse?

_____
_____
_____
_____

What are some of the different legitimate places where you can look for a horse?
What are the problems with purchasing a horse from a 'kill pen'?

Even your mentor does not have x-ray vision! Why is a pre-purchase exam important?
What will the pre-purchase exam tell you?
And what will it not tell you?

_____
_____
_____
_____

How much can you spend to buy a horse?

How much will you spend on routine needs, like board, feed, veterinarian and farrier care, and lessons?

Why must you get a signed contract?

_____
_____
_____
_____
_____
_____
_____
_____
_____
_____

"I was drawn to horses as if they were magnets. It must be genetic. It makes horse people different from everyone else. It divides humanity into those who love horses and those who simply don't know how."

~Allan J. Hamilton

BUT WAIT! THERE'S MORE! YOUR PROFESSIONAL SUPPORT TEAM

Along with your horse care team (at your barn of choice) there is a host of other professionals you will rely on for the health, safety, and comfort of your horse.

The first of these is your veterinarian. The barn may have a relationship in place that gets you great service, or you may have to make your own arrangements. Your horse will receive both "well-baby" care like vaccinations, deworming, and an annual check up. And you will also want to have a great relationship with your veterinarian in the case of injury of illness leading to urgent care.

It helps for you to have a basic knowledge of signs and symptoms. So there are some things your should learn about.

How do you take the vital signs of your horse?
How do you identify the signs of colic, abscesses, and other common ailments?
Where is your first aid kit (human and equine)?
Do you know basic first aid for your horse?
If not, how are you going to learn it?

What are the recommended vaccines for your area?
What deworming protocol does your veterinarian recommend?
Who is your veterinarian?
What is the basic annual care package your veterinarian recommends?
What are the special needs of your horse (these may have been revealed in your pre-purchase exam)?
How does my veterinarian expect to be paid?

MY VET PLAN

_____

_____

_____

How often does your horse see a farrier?
What are any special needs for farrier care?
How does my farrier expect to be paid?

MY FARRIER PLAN

_____

_____

How often does your horse see a dentist?
What is your schedule for saddle fitting?

_____

_____

INSURANCE AND POWERS OF ATTORNEY: PROTECTING YOURSELF AND YOUR HORSES

The purpose of insurance for your horse is to spread risk, and its related financial considerations, over time. You need to know what your threshold for self-insurance is. In other words, how much money do you have set aside to pay for emergency veterinary bills, or to replace your horse if it dies. These concerns are covered by equine life insurance and major medical. Your insurance plan should also have coverage for liability and personal property damage.

What sort of insurance coverage do you have for your horse, yourself, and your equine property?

What sort of medical coverage do you have for your horse?

Can you afford major veterinary expenses for your horse without insurance?

How much liability insurance do you have that covers incidents with your horse?

Is your personal property (tack, equipment, bridles, etc.) covered by insurance?

Have you taken a photo inventory of all of your personal property?

Who has your power of attorney to make decisions about your horse if you cannot?
Do the people who are involved with the care of your horse know who has the POA? Your veterinarian? Barn or stable owner? Riding partner? Spouse? Instructor? Horse trainer?

END OF LIFE PLAN

_____
_____
_____
_____
_____
_____
_____
_____
_____
_____
_____
_____

Are you prepared to make the decision to put your horse down?
What are the factors that play into your decision to put your horse down?
What are the "quality of life" and safety issues involved in making that decision?
What memorials can you make to remember your horse?

What is the End of Life Plan for my beloved horse..

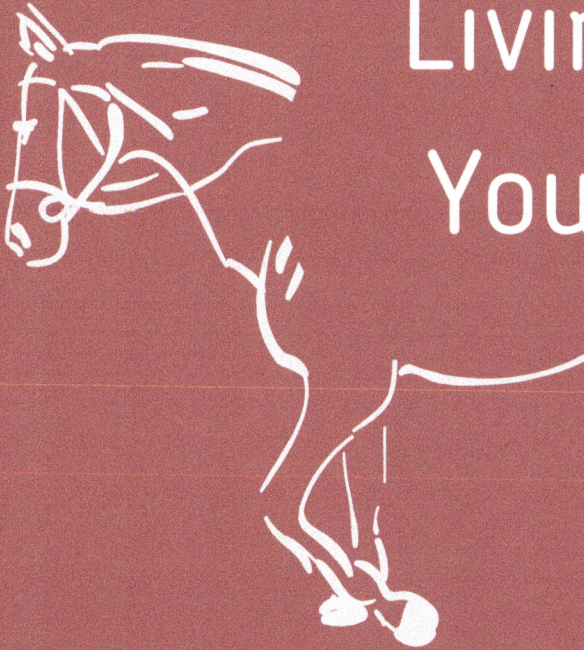

PART SIX

Living With
Your Horse

YOUR OWN PLACE: A HOME ON THE RANGE

For many ladies of a certain age living with your horse in your own backyard is the high point of your horse dreams. This might be the right path for you if you are approaching retirement. You have no more daily family or job obligations. Your finances are sound. Your health is good.

Successful "horse at home" people have experienced the hard reality check on the amount of time, energy, physical demands, money and education involved in this choice.

Here are some questions to guide your reality check:

Why do you want to have your own place instead of boarding your horse?

What are the most important things you need at your own place?

What are the prices for farms in your area?

Which of the daily routine and chores around a barn do you do now?
How does the change of seasons affect your ability to do those chores?
Do you have help with doing the daily routine?
Can you do them without that help? Can you find someone else to help if your current assistant is unable to do so?

Does doing the chores cut into the time you spend actually riding or training or otherwise enjoying your horse?

Are you working with a real estate professional with experience in farms and equine properties?
What are the benefits and drawbacks of 'equine residential communities'?
What about 'shared community living?'

If you are considering moving to another area, what research are you doing?
What are the most important considerations for moving?

In addition to a friendly horse environment, what other things are important for you?

What is the medical care like?
What cultural and social activities are important to you?
What about churches and other religious and spiritual activities?
What is the general political climate of the area?
What are the shopping opportunities?

Do you enjoy a community with many different cultures and ethnicities or do you prefer familiar settings and people?

What services does the area have for an aging population?

Now that you have done the research, what is your plan?

_____
_____
_____
_____
_____
_____
_____
_____
_____

"It is not selfish to love yourself, take care of yourself, and make your happiness a priority. It's necessary."

~Mandy Hale

BOARDERS: BENEFIT OR BOTHER

If you are convinced that your "horse at home" plan is sound, then a next logical step is to decide if you also want to grow your own community by having boarders on your property. This gets you into a whole new space of owning a running (however small or large) a horse business. If people pay you to keep their horse, even if you build it like a co-op, there are specific legal, tax, and insurance ramifications.

What are the options you can offer for boarders?
How much extra work will a boarder add to your workload and take away from your time with your horse?
How will you deal with a boarder who pays late or not at all?
What are the legal options open to you?
What are the details of your boarding contract?
What are your barn rules? (There are links to sample contracts and rules on the website.)
What kind of insurance do you have to protect yourself and your property?
How will you 'fire' a difficult boarder? What your your legal options?

_____

_____

_____

_____

_____

BARN FIRES, NATURAL DISASTERS, AND EVACUATIONS

Here we are looking at the events we hope NEVER happen.
As with most things a bit of prevention will contribute to your peaceful life, so even though some subjects are tough to think about, its a really good idea to have a plan.

When was the last time your local fire department examined your barn and property?
What steps have you taken to follow their recommendations?
What steps do you take if there is a barn fire?

What condition is your electrical system?

What are the warning signs of spontaneous combustion?
What steps do you take if you think this is imminent?
What is the checklist for an evacuation? (Hint: P. 182 of Riders of a Certain Age, or the website)
What is the most important step you can take to prepare for an evacuation?

How do you prepare for a hurricane?

How can you prepare for a wildfire?
What are the steps to take when your horse has been exposed to smoke or fire?

How can you prepare your property and horses for a tornado?
What can you do to protect yourself when a tornado approaches?
What should you do after a tornado hits?

What should you do in the fall to prepare your property and horses for blizzards and ice storms?

What are the dangers of space heaters?

Commit your Evacuation plan to writing (then print it off and post it in your barn so any guests, family members, or helpers can read it in the case of an emergency)

_____

_____

_____

_____

_____

_____

_____

_____

_____

ON THE ROAD: MONEY, MEDICINE, AND PRACTICALITIES

Some horse owners want to combine their recreation with horses and their recreational vehicle to live the life of a nomad. One of my favorite veterinarians retired, sold her home, and loaded up two dogs, a cat, her partner, and a nice pair of trail-riding horses, and off they went. I follow their adventures on Facebook! If this is your dream then preparation is important before you ride off into the sunset.

What does your "travel with horses" dream look like?

_____

_____

Why do you want to live on the road with your horse?
What research have you done to find the details of living on the road?
What actions have you taken to make sure you are safe living on the road?
Who can you work with to learn the basics of your truck, trailer, and LQ maintenance and repairs?

_____

_____

_____

Riders of a certain age need to make special plans for their own health as well as their horse's.

How are you preparing yourself to deal with your physical needs on the road?
What kind of steps can you take if you need a doctor or a prescription refill on the road?

More "dot the i's and cross the t's" details:

What have you done to simplify managing your finances while on the road?
Where can you find the residency and driver's license requirements for states where you might be staying for any length of time?
How can you prepare your horse for a long trip?
Where can you find a veterinarian when you are on the road?
How can you plan your trip to make it as comfortable for you and your horse as possible?
How far can you travel in a day?

What is the travel plan for your journey?

_____
_____
_____
_____
_____
_____
_____
_____
_____
_____
_____
_____
_____
_____
_____
_____

How can you determine if your horse is comfortable?
Which roadside assistance companies do you know?
Where can you find information about accommodations while traveling?

_____

_____

_____

_____

_____

"Women grow radical with age. One day an army of gray-haired women may quietly take over the earth."

~Fran Severn

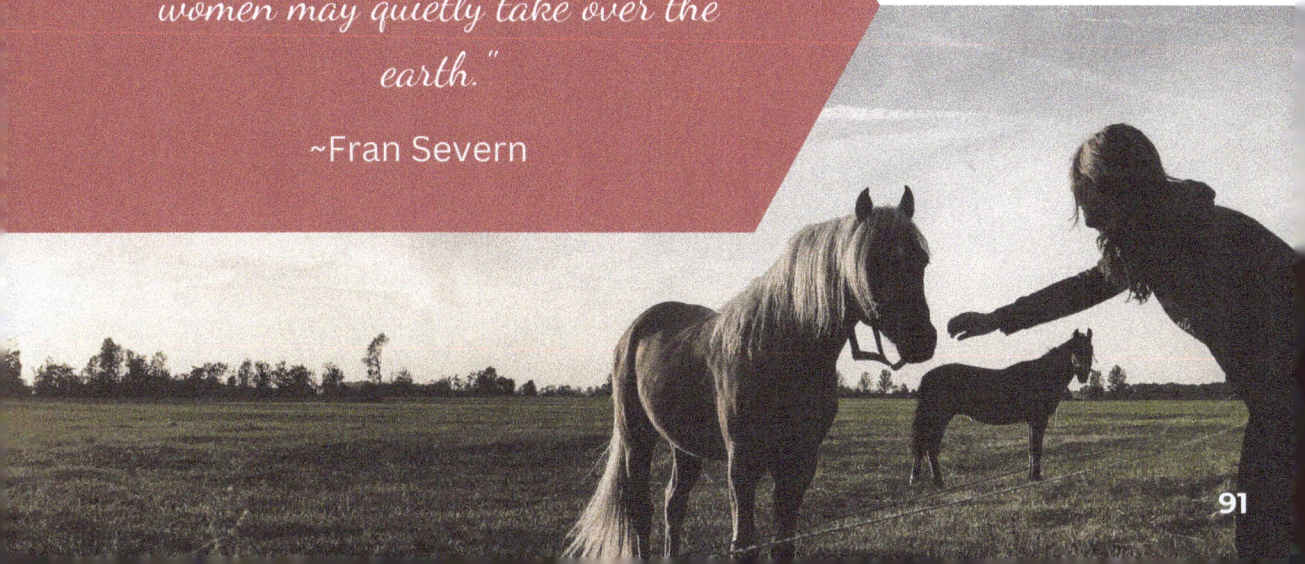

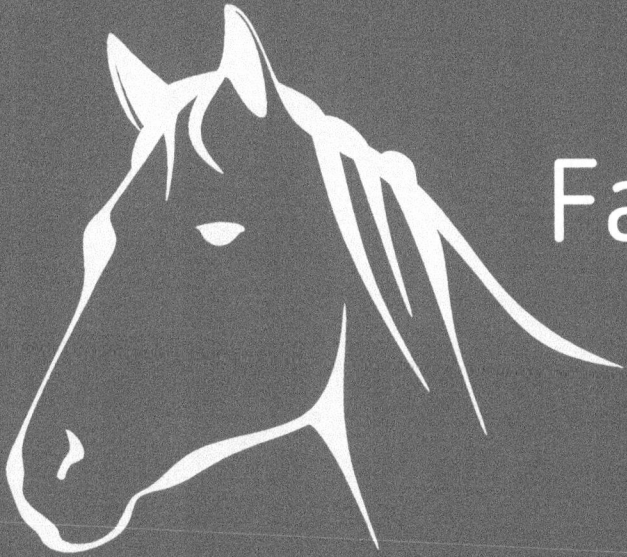

PART SEVEN

Family And Finances

MONEY AND MANURE

If you want to have this manure-making experience, you have to know where the money is coming from! It's part of being a good steward for your horse hobby and protects your family as well. In fact, careful consideration of finances (even if we would rather scrub out a slimy water bucket than balance our checkbook) is the best way to gain support from your loved ones for the hobby you love.

It's time to review your monthly and annual budget. (A link to a good chart for determining your spending is on the RidersofaCertainAge website.)
Use this chart to get a realistic look at your income and expenses.

What expenses are vital and unavoidable?

_____

_____

What expenses are optional?

_____

_____

Go through your bills, receipts, and credit cards and identify those things that you can live without (how many streaming services?

_____

_____

_____

How often do you eat out or order in?)

_____

_____

_____

_____

Make an appointment with a financial planner to review your current state of finances and plan for the next 10-20 years. What are the biggest concerns and how can you plan for them?

How much do you have in savings and investments?

If the economy crashes how will you adjust?

If you are still working, what are the chances that you will be 'downsized' or forced to leave because of your age? (It's not legal, but it happens.)

If you are offered early retirement or a severance package, will you compensate for your lost income?

What are the possibilities of finding another job?
Will another job come with benefits?

Is your company solvent, as far as you know?

_____

_____

_____

_____

_____

_____

_____

Do you own your house and, if so, how much equity do you have?

Can you take out a home equity loan and comfortably repay it with your current income?

Can you do so if your income is reduced?

Do you have a second income?
How important is that to your family finances?
 Is it critical or is it used for optional activities and purchases?

Do you use that income for savings for retirement or major expenses (new roof on the house, replacing aging appliances)?

_____

_____

_____

_____

_____

_____

What is your medical converage?
How can you pay for the things that are not covered?

Do you have 'catastrophic' insurance? This covers things like long-term care and rehabilitation.

_____

_____

DEALING WITH AN UNSUPPORTIVE SPOUSE

At the beginning of this fabulous journey we talked about our own passion for horses. And we understand that horse people are their own kind of crazy, not easily understood by folks who aren't horsepeople. If you are married to, or live your life with someone who is not a horse person, you can't expect them to just always get on your game plan. You have to play fair.

So it makes a lot of sense for you to seek to understand their point of view. Life will be easier for you when you do.

How does your partner feel about your passion for horses?
If you both enjoy horses, what are the things that you do together?
Do you ride or belong to a riding group?
If not a rider, does he show support in other ways: helping at the stable, driving the trailer, going to shows?

_____

_____

_____

_____

_____

_____

_____

If your partner does not share your enthusiasm, how does he show that?

Does your partner have his own hobbies and activities?

What are they?

Do you share any of them?

If you don't share any of them, how do you support him in his interests?

_____

_____

_____

_____

_____

_____

Do you have mutual friends who share your interests?

Is your partner also approaching retirement and dealing with the many changes in his life and routine?

How is he reacting to these changes?

How does the conversation go when you talk about this next stage in his life, in your lives?

_____

_____

_____

If your partner is unsupportive, how do you talk about it?

What happens when you try to open a conversation?
Can you find ways to compromise on your interests?
What ways can you find to do that?

_____

_____

_____

_____

_____

_____

Complaints about horses interfering with your relationship are usually a symptom, not a cause. Would you consider visiting a counselor, with or without your spouse?

_____

_____

_____

_____

_____

PROTECTING YOUR HORSE WHEN YOU ARE GONE

A few years back I had the honor to support a family member with a terminal diagnosis. It's not the most pleasant of situations. But as we age so do our family and friends and eventually, someone has to serve. In this case, careful preparations were made for the long-term care of every animal and her horses came to live with me when she passed away.

This is an area where pre-planning is important so that everything runs smoothly. You not only need to plan. You also need to incorporate your plan for your horse's care into your documents and make sure that the people implementing your plan know your wishes.

Do you have a plan for taking care of your horses if you are unable to do so?

Who will take care of your horse(s)?
Have you discussed it with them and are they willing and able to do so?

_____
_____
_____
_____
_____
_____
_____
_____
_____

Have you talked about the financial aspects of caring for your horses and made arrangements for that?

Are the others involved in caring for your horse: stable owner if you board, farrier, veterinarian, etc. aware of your plans?

_____

_____

_____

_____

_____

_____

_____

_____

Final Thoughts

So here we are!

We've gone from being individuals with a passion for horses to joining together as a community of horsewomen. It's been a journey.

We've read about building our lives around horses, thought deeply about what that means for each of us, and shared those insights with each other. We shared our stories, shared our hopes, shared our dreams.

We laughed at the silly things we've done and at the funny and sometimes unbelievable things our horses have done. And sometimes we've cried. Cried at the inevitable heartbreak that comes with loving those big, gentle, mystical, sadly not-immortal creatures. Because that's part of what love is. We've learned from each other and from our horses.

And the journey never ends. As long as hoof meets ground and large dark eyes look into ours and give us glimpses into their souls, the journey continues.

Stay with us. Stay with your group, your sisterhood.

Never let our journey together end.

Fran